Alcohol

Aversion Therapy

by E. Nuff & S. Topp

Alcohol   **Aversion   Therapy**

Are you addicted to alcohol? Sick of thinking about it all the time? Is it ruining your life, your health and/or your relationships? Ready to kick the habit and get your life back? Tried everything to stop?

Finally, here is a way to help you help yourself give up for good. This Alcohol Aversion Therapy book is designed to really put you off it. A series of absolutely revolting pictures to turn off that old desire for the unhealthy. Read the instructions carefully, as the method aims to combine several processes to help you free yourself from wanting or needing alcohol ever again. You have strong willpower. Remember a time when you used it and bring it into play to assist this Aversion Therapy Book.

Copyright: © S J Quast 2016
Photographs Copyright © S J Quast 2016

ISBN-13: 978-1539043041
ISBN-10: 1539043045

IMPORTANT:

read the last 3 pages first.

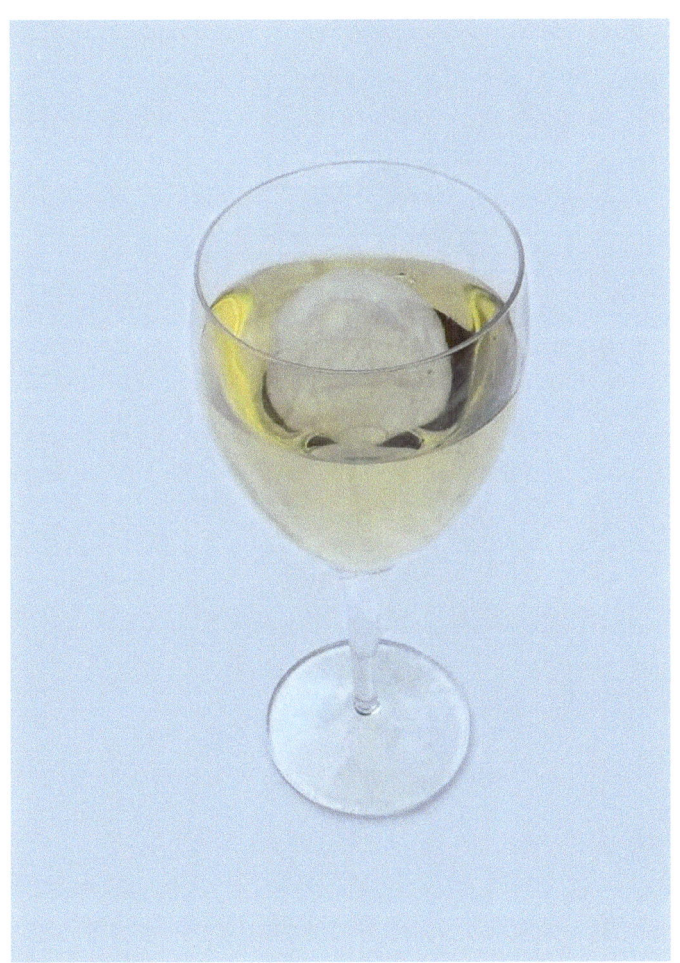

Eeeeek!

Mealy worms!

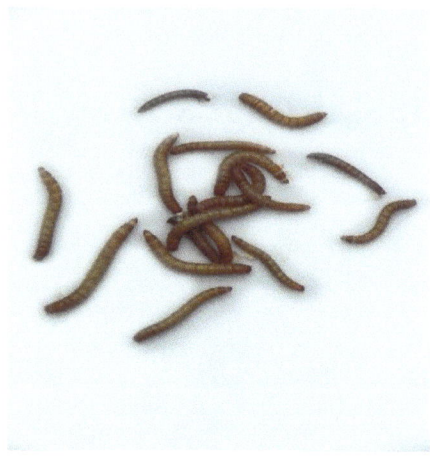

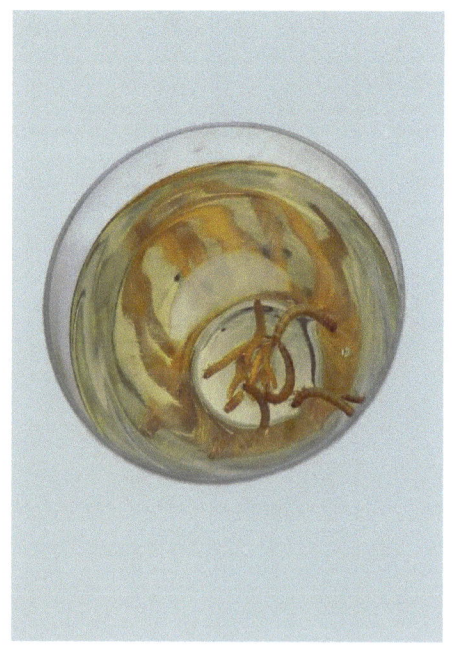

YUCKY!

Wine with mealy worms....

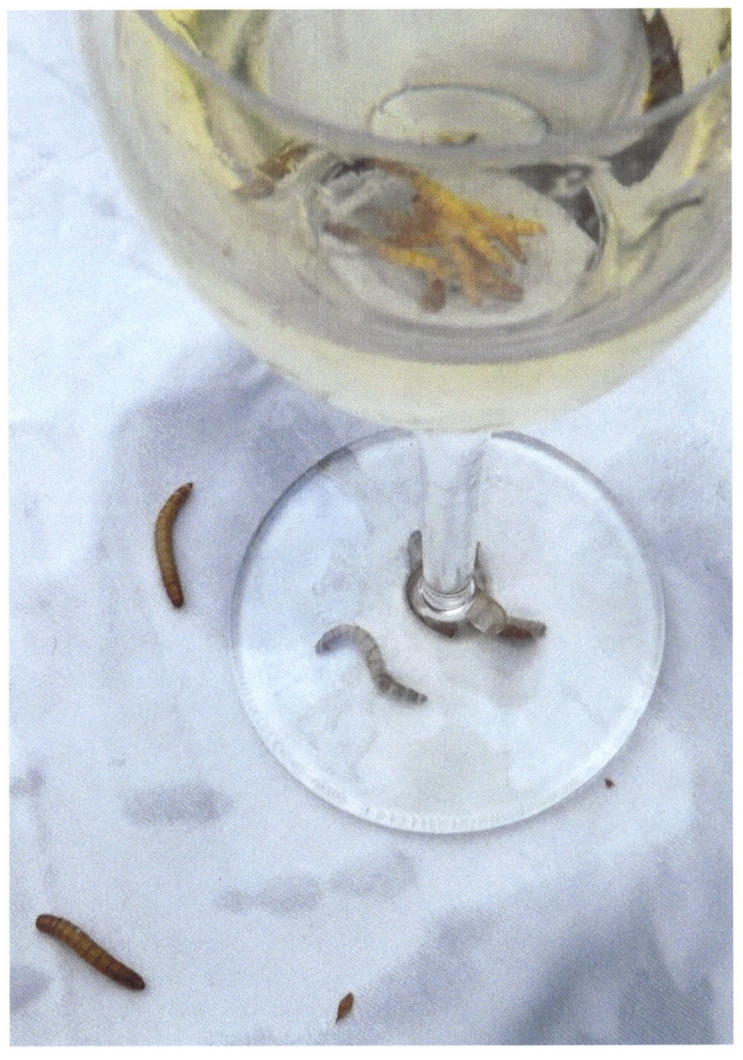

They wriggle. Errrrk!
Ruined. Revolting!

SPEW!

Remember how it feels, smells, tastes
BEFORE you drink....
and just drink WATER instead.

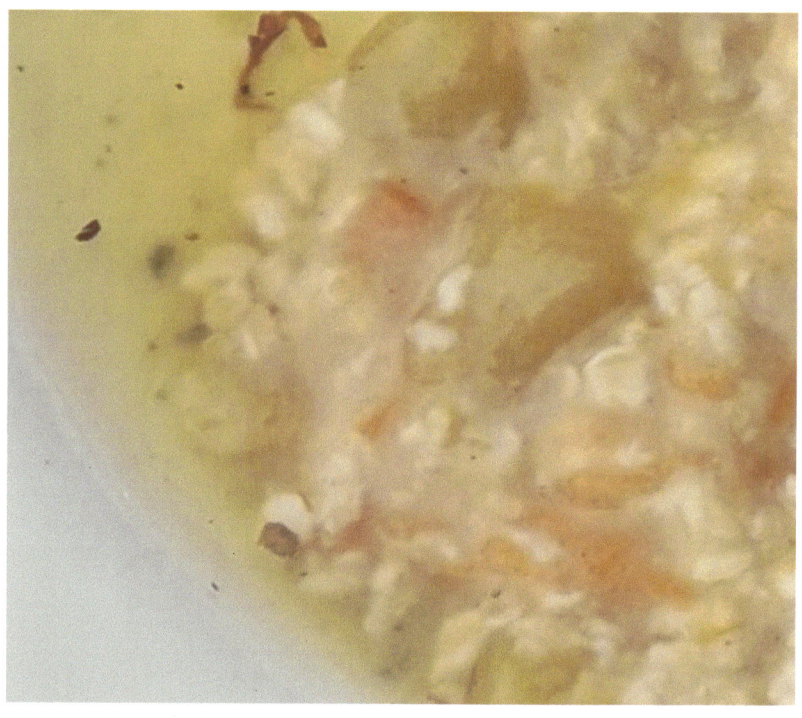

Be reminded of slimy vomit every time you
think about drinking alcohol. Remember
the taste and smell. URRGGH!

CHERK!

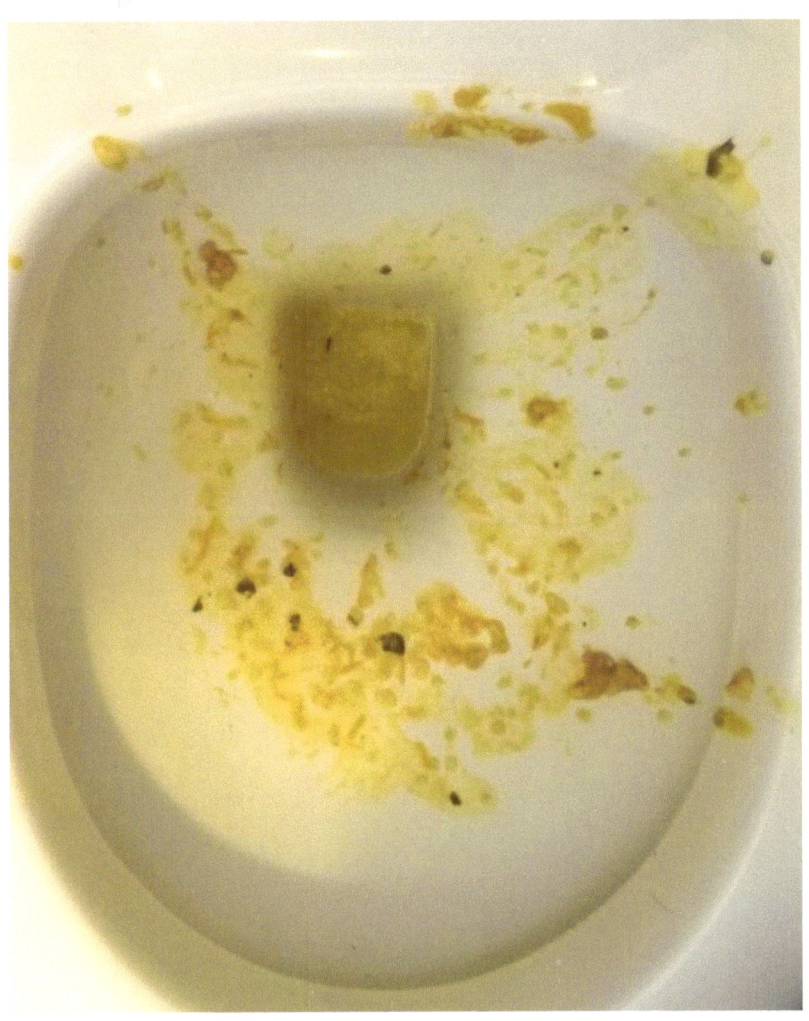

How many times has a night of drinking ended like this?

Cigarettes, alcohol, VOMIT

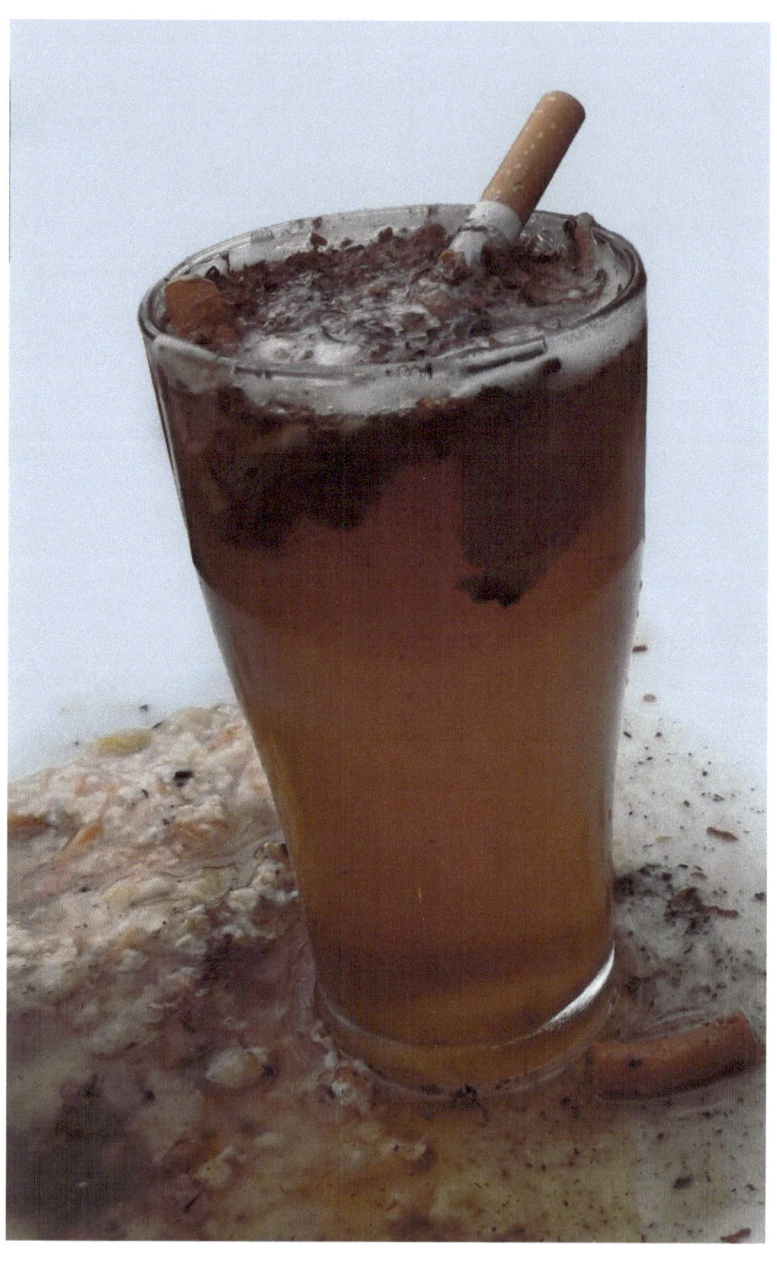

Alcohol can turn reality into a drunken haze. What is the focus of your life?

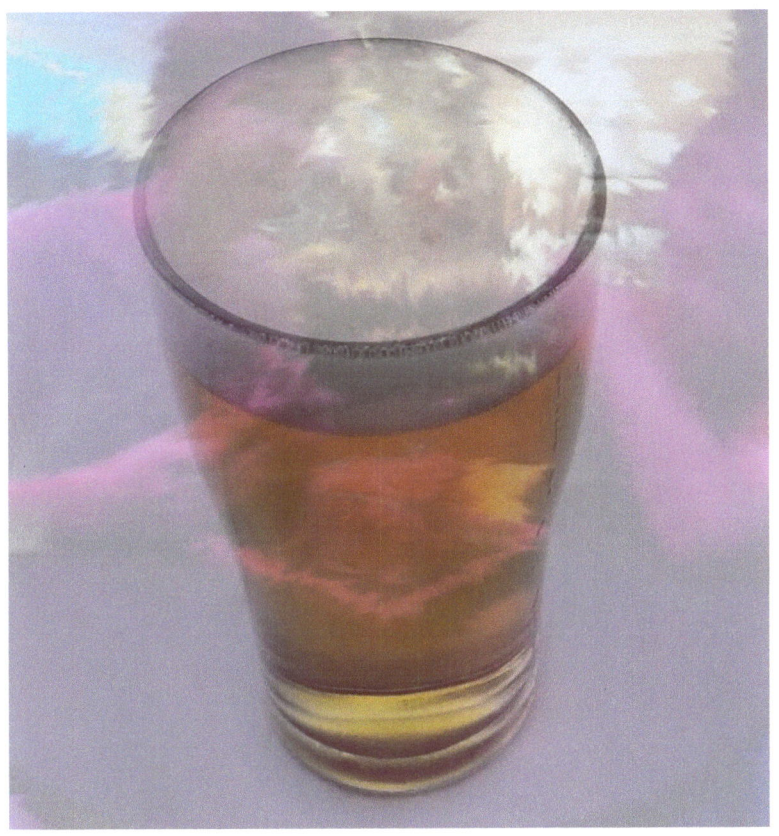

Enjoy life without alcohol to make the most of your friends, food and memories. If you can't face life without it ... perhaps you should see a counsellor ... and make adjustments to your attitude so that you CAN enjoy life sober.

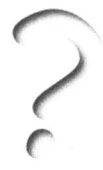

So what DID happen that night?

Who did you meet?

What did you say?

Uuuuurr
    rrrr
        rrghhh!

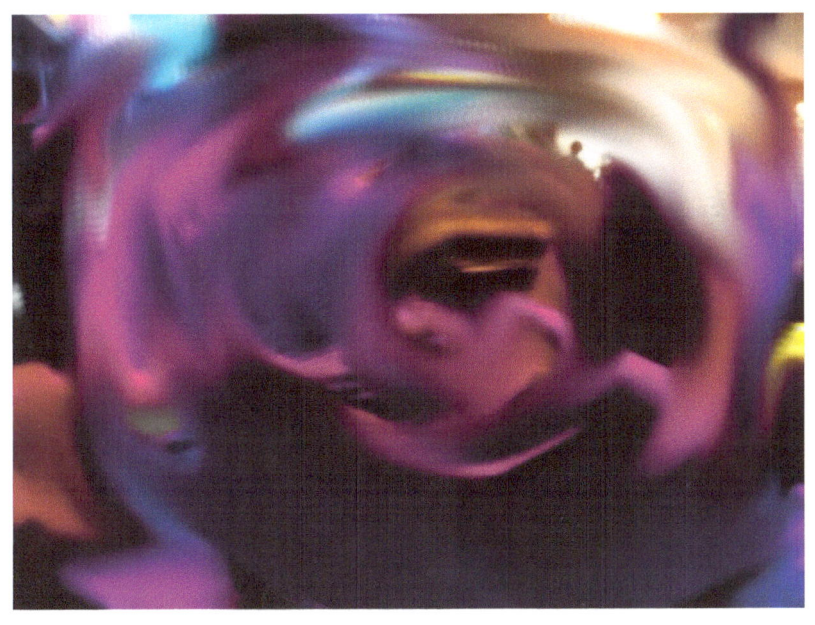

Limit regrets,
improve memory: Stay sober

Urrck! You know what that smells like! Putrid. Od Ash. Acrid vomit. Making you want to gag and retch. You know what it feels like. Slimy and sticky. You know what it tastes like.

It reminds you of that alcohol you used to drink. It can kill. It attacks the kidneys, liver, brain. You are intelligent. Use your intelligence and stay that way.

Be glad you have decided not to overindulge any more. You are freeing yourself from that old alcohol habit. Stop the cycle. Drink water. Imagine it soothing and relaxing you. It can.

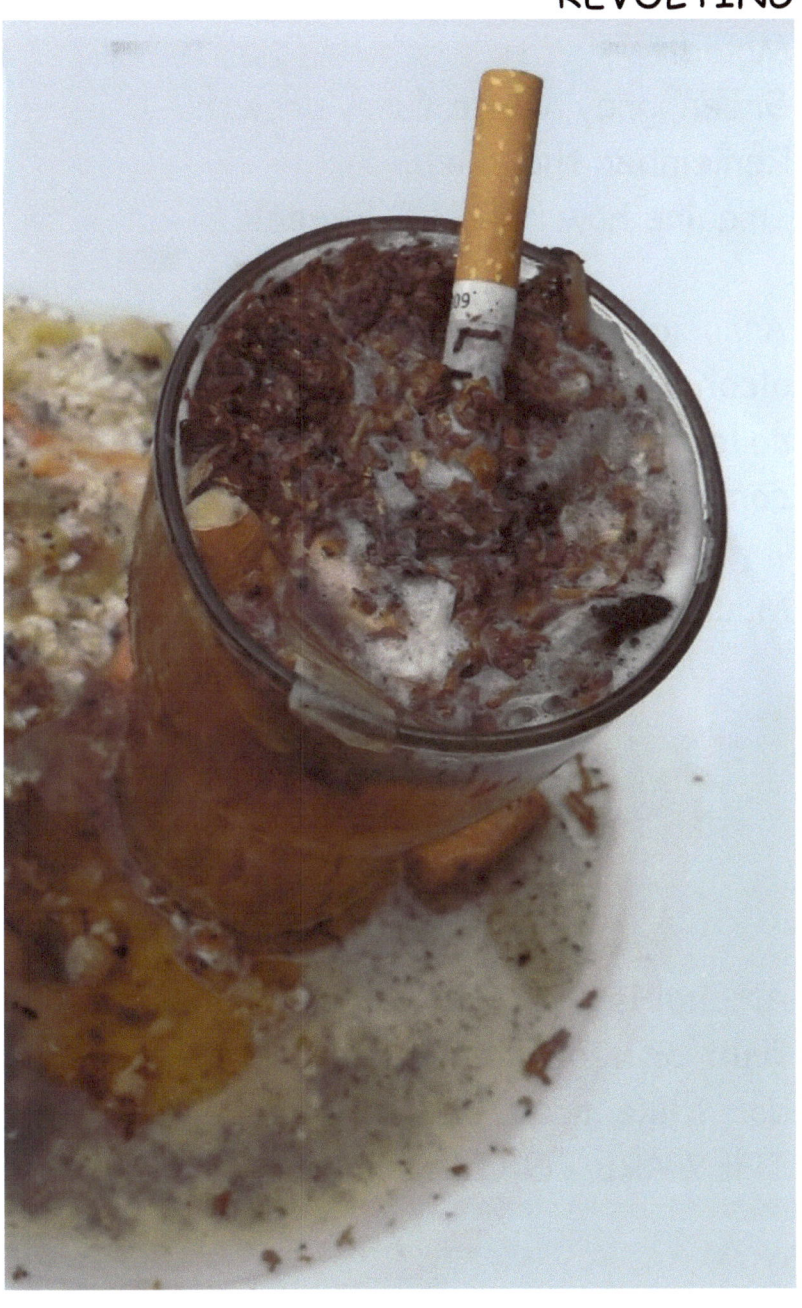

URRGH!
Mould!
Green, grey, white furry growth.
Remember the smell.
Imagine how it feels. Eeeeek!

Associate that smell and feel with bringing alcohol to your lips. That is one thing you no longer want to do ever again. Safely and comfortably avoid alcohol and mould.

Mouldy bread?
    Mouldy grapes?
        Mouldy hops?
            Mouldy potatoes?
                Mouldy fruit?

Alcohol is a by-product of mouldy and off fruit or vegetables. There is a reason we don't like mould or its by-products ...
THEY ARE TOXIC !

URRGH!

Mould !

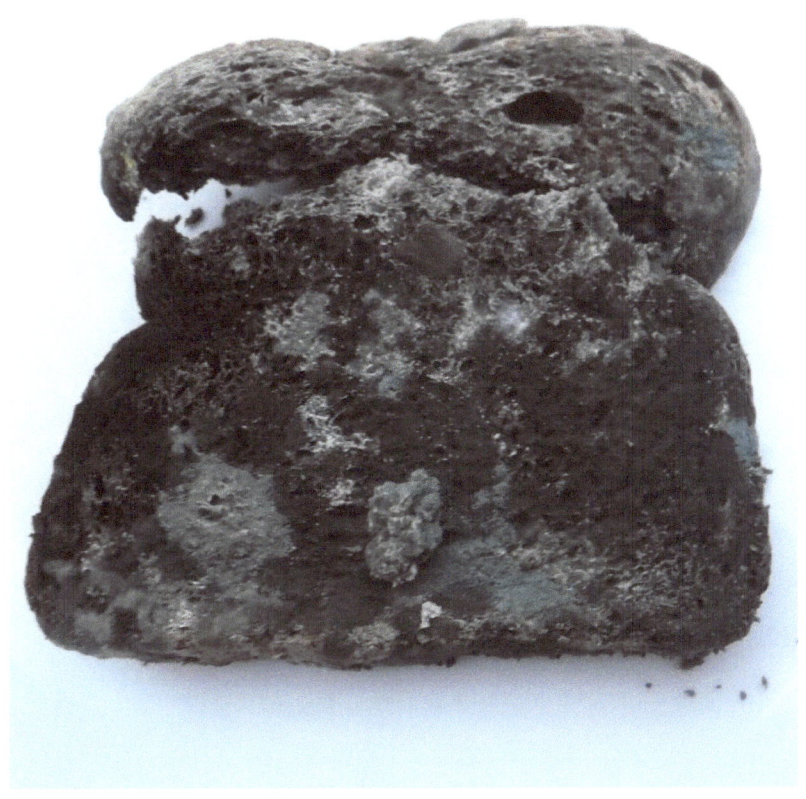

mouldy/fermented => alcohol
NO THANKS

SHIT.   Keep booze out of your body

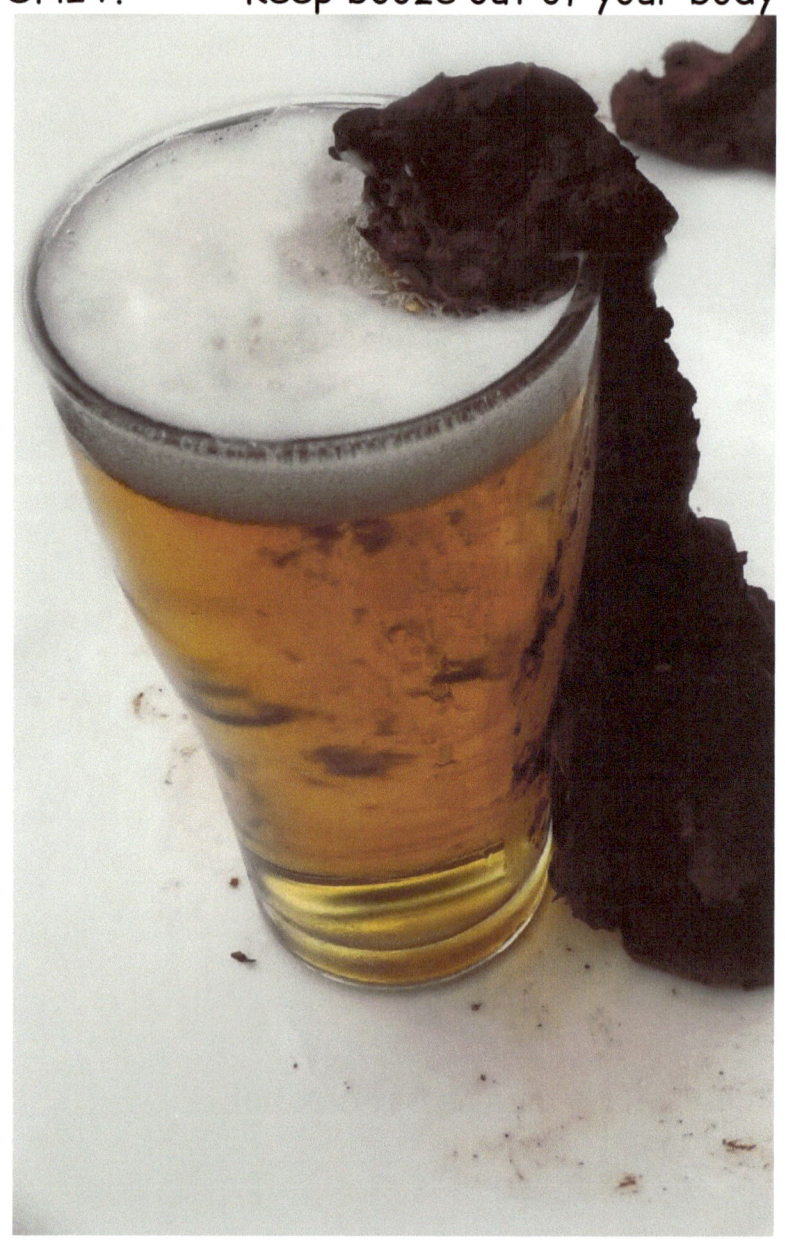

Poo.

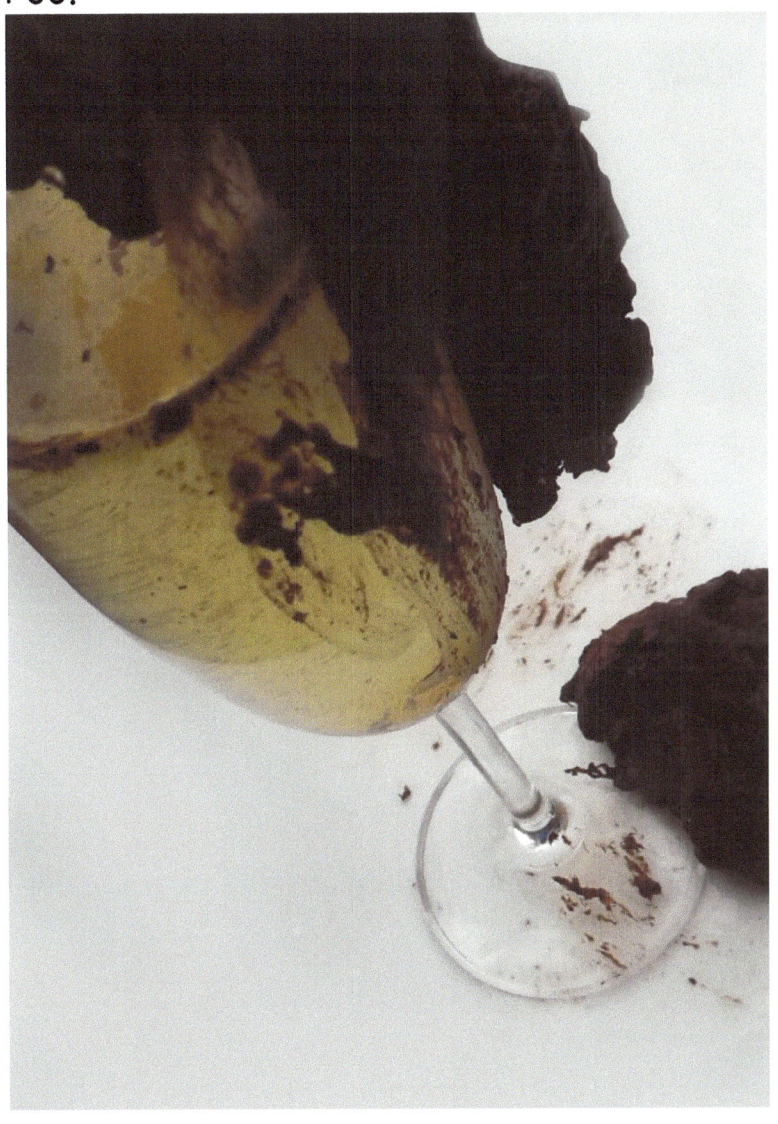

Let alcohol bypass your body.
Better just tip it straight down the loo.

Yuck, YUCK!   May all alcohol taste like ashtray.

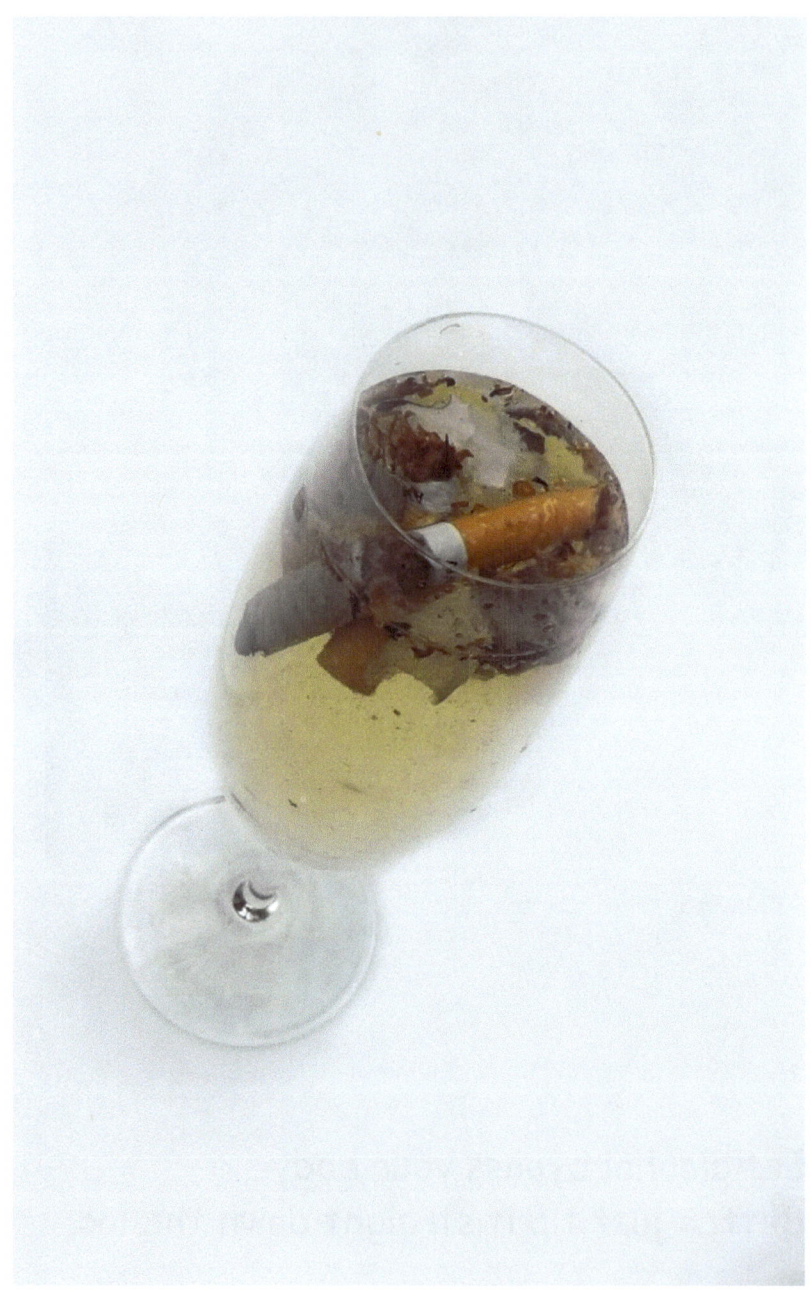

Wooohaarrr

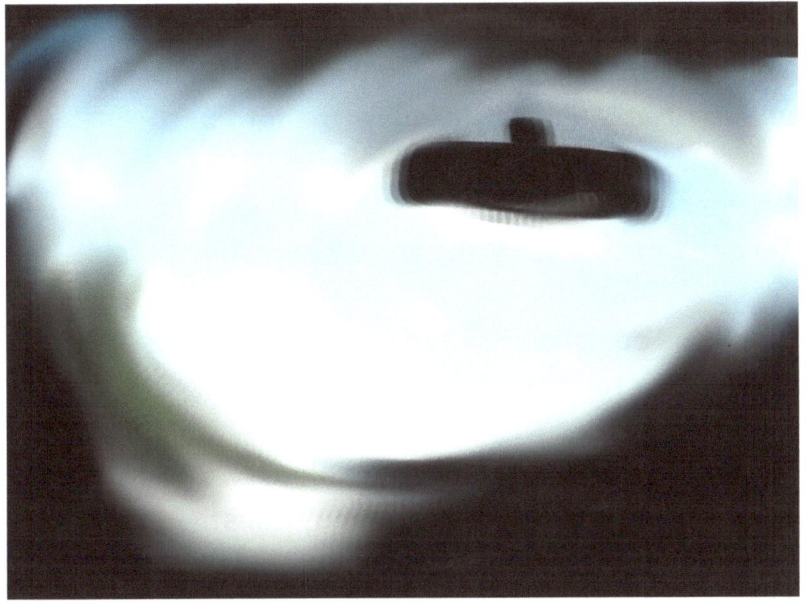

How many times have you driven under the influence?

Glad you didn't get booked? Should you have been?

How terrible would it be if you had killed someone?

How awful would it be if you had killed a loved-one?

You kill their respect for you when you get pissed.

Perhaps you used to drown your sorrows with alcohol. It just made it worse. You no longer need to do that. Just breathe deeply, drink water, relax, go for a walk.

You can let unwanted thoughts flow away. Thoughts are not facts unless you allow them to be.

If there is alcohol in the house, lock it away and forget where it is. Make it difficult to access.

Keep this book handy when you go to the store. Bypass the liquor store.

We are mostly water and get thirsty when we need more. Alcohol doesn't quench thirst. Drink only water.

Value your body and only put good things in it. Drink water.

Love yourself. You are worth it.

STOP flushing your life away!

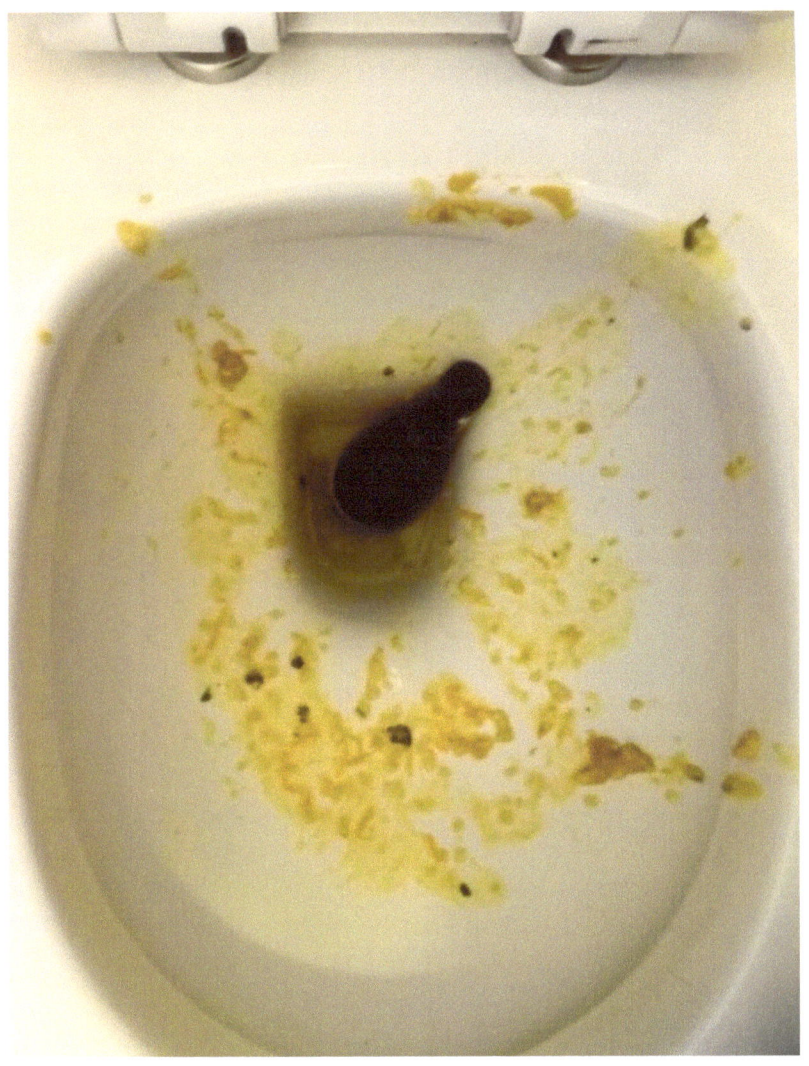

Alcohol is SHIT !

Instructions:

Are you ready to stop drinking alcohol? If you really want to get rid of that old addiction you will need:

1. this book.

2. something that *smells* bad to YOU (e.g. rotten egg, rancid oil, off milk, diluted cleaning product, rotten garbage or compost, etc).

3. (optional) something that *tastes* bad to YOU personally or e.g. smelly goats cheese, over-ripe bananas, Tabasco sauce, whatever turns you off.

PROCEDURE

First:
Look at the picture of the alcohol on the first page. Note how much you would want to drink it (on a scale from 1 to 10).

Second:
Put the food you hate in your mouth and smell the substance that revolts you while looking at the rest of the pictures in the book. Spend at least a minute on each of the pictures you find revolting. Read. Imagine a better life free of that old addiction.

Third:
Look at the first picture again and notice how little you need it now (on a scale of 1 to 10).

Fourth:
Keep the book with you when you go shopping to remind yourself to connect alcohol with aversion. Don't buy any.

Fifth:

Remember to **PAUSE:**

Punch the air 100 times or go for a walk etc. at times when you used to drink alcohol. This is to pause and avoid that revolting toxin. You can get a good feeling from exercise instead.

Air can be breathed in deeply to relax you and fill you with energy and evaporate those old cravings. Imagine stress leaving you as you exhale.

Understand that water can be drunk to wash away any future shadows of cravings. You are often only thirsty for water when you think you want to drink alcohol.

Select better, healthier drinks. Water, tea or even coffee.

Ensure that alcohol is difficult to access: locked away or unavailable. Ideally, don't keep any. Tip it down the sink.

Welcome to a new life where you have control over those old addictions you used to have. You can remember to live free of alcohol.

Disclaimer: no guarantees given for effectiveness. Pictures are planned to supplement the effect of an existing desire to stop drinking alcohol, and help you to help yourself reduce cravings for it. Use common sense when selecting substances that smell or taste bad to supplement the therapy. Ensure they are safe, non-toxic and non-allergenic. When in doubt consult your counsellor or doctor.

The End   =>   the first day of the rest of your life